This is dedicated to my mom and my grandmother, who never gave up on me.

Nursing Rants

I had so many journal entries from my first year working as an RN, that I decided I wanted to share this experience with nurses around the world. I omit the name of the nightmare hospital, of course. I also don't name any patients or identifiers, but I believe I've mentioned just enough to give you the gist.

I did have my license suspended for a year, and no work. I felt as though I had hit rock bottom and would never recover from it. So this is for those of you who feel as though you're risking your license and everything you have worked so hard to achieve. This is for those who have already lost their license, or had trouble with The Board. And finally it's for everyone who just likes to hear a good rant.

"If you want a picture of the future, imagine a boot stamping on a human face—for ever."

-George Orwell -*1984*

Chapter 1

My First Job as an RN!

March, 2013

Upon graduating from nursing school, I applied to take my NCLEX. I wondered why it was taking so long for the BON to send me my ATT, so I called them.

They had lost my transcripts.

After re-ordering them at the cost of $22, I was set. I passed the exam on my first try, and I was now a registered nurse!

It was March 15, 2013... two years to the day since I lost my beloved grandmother.

Something about this damn date.

I had applied to about 40 jobs since graduating and only got 3 call-backs. While I was still in nursing school, the job offers all said "6 months' experience," but naturally upon graduating, that changed to one year.

No sweat. I'll find something.

The first call I get is from the hospital an hour away from me, for inpatient rehab. The guy has my resume and sees that I was an unpaid care-taker prior to starting nursing school. It was my grandmother. There was nothing more important to me than her. He knew this, yet called me in for a 2-hour interview. We got along well and I could tell he liked me, but then he introduced me to Mother Hen. The veteran nurse who's been in the game since the 70's and "doesn't like new grads." I didn't stand a chance with her.

The next call was at the *same hospital* but different floor. And the third call was at the *same hospital*, different floor. Hmmm...

I took the second offer.

The interview: This is at an inner city hospital right in the middle of *everything*. I walk onto the floor and immediately sense the overwhelming anxiety. The smell of shit and body stank is incredible. The lights are asepticized, bright & unwelcoming. The color scheme is the opposite of warm and the whole floor looks like it hasn't been redesigned since the 80's (broken counter top at nurse's station, holes in the wall, etc.). There's a simple explanation for this: the hospital cannot ever shut this floor down for renovations because this floor is the other floors' bitch.

The nurses are harried and there's sooooooo many people! It's like something I'd see on t.v., in NYC or some place with a high population. I could tell that the Nurse Supervisor was a bitch as soon as I met her. A bitch to other people yes, but I liked her. Maybe she'd had to be a bitch in her life, who knows. The charge nurse took me around and told me in an eerie tone, "We looOOoove new grads!" This should've been my cue to turn around and never come back.

But I was desperate. I took the job. Post-operative floor, or so I thought.

If only I'd have trusted my gut & walked away.

* * *

His Name is Mud

April, 2013

I got an admit from The Sticks the other day. He's a relatively young 40-something, being rolled onto the floor, and he looks quiet and calm. I introduce myself to him and get him set up nicely in his bed, taking into account his declaration of severe pain (these always scare me, 'cause you just never know...).

I study his chart more in depth and consult 2 residents on the matter, as we have no idea what's causing his pain. All we know is that it's in his abdomen.

Before long, that quiet & calm new admit begins to get restless about his pain (what I was afraid of). In my first month as a new nurse, I've already been exposed to episodes like this. There is literally nothing I can do at the moment, as the 2 docs are in the office reviewing this man's tests. I know this will go sour real fast, I just know it.

And sure enough, it does. He starts insulting me in the hallway, & then he hurls his IV pole at me.

I'm always liked by people, even the worst kinds of people. I'm placid & not an assertive person, nor do I attract drama or misery in my life. Still being new on the floor, I can feel frequent occurrences like this will drive me over the edge, & I'm afraid I'll quit or have a stroke. After all, I didn't become a cop or security guard now, did I?

I lose my temper & tell him that I cannot prescribe, that's the Doctors' role. I walk out of his room visibly upset, & tell the Charge Nurse to reassign me, which she does.

Guess what. Next day, who is my patient?

Yep!

Dealing with daily trials such as these has done fried my nerves, and at this point I am sure that I don't like this job. Sure it can be a character builder, and in the long run I will more calmly deal with such cases. In other words, it'll make me a stronger nurse.

But I can't help but feel ever-so nauseated each morning when I wake up & prepare for the hour-long drive into the city. Because this is a hit-the-ground-running type of place. From the surface, the patients, their families, and of course the employees can see that it's a poorly managed floor. I don't think this is good for a new nurse, but unfortunately as a new nurse, we can't be picky.

Needless to say, the patient apologized to me & we went about our lives.

* * *

What Caused my Patient to Become Psychotic?

May, 2013

Keep in mind that I am still in orientation.

I am given a 60-something male patient who is accusing everybody of trying to kill him. His wife is at the bedside and she is terribly worried about him acting out of character. I keep pushing the big D into his IV, as he has a spinal injury & is visibly in pain. But the big D is all I can give him.

I call the doctor to see if we can change to mild pain pills. I just have a hunch that the Dilaudid is making him act this way. I tell his wife of my plan and she agrees with it.

I go to another patient's room to learn about her brain injury, when of course like it does every 3 minutes, my phone rings. I can't hear the person on the other end as the nurse is teaching me and doesn't seem to notice (or care) that I have a phone call, & the floor I work on is always loud & frantic. When the teaching's done I walk out into the hallway, and everybody's running around like crazy. The Code Green notice is blaring on the intercom and my heart goes into overdrive (that's a psych emergency).

When I go back into my 60-something patient's room, all the nurses are at his bed holding him down. The bed is elevated as high as it can go, and in reverse

Trendelenburg. Did I mention my patient's completely naked? In a semi-private room.

I find out he's just had a psychotic break, but I knew from his chart & speaking to his wife that he had no psych history. So we give him something to calm him down, at which point I notice that his labs show that he's positive for Hep C. It turns out he and his wife already knew this, so how come none of us staff did? I felt once again that I'd somehow dropped the ball. I'm a bad nurse for letting this happen and I deserve to be stripped of my license.

I get him adjusted to the pain pills, which work wonders for him. His wife requests me back the following 2 days, and I get to see him make a full recovery. Before I discharge him we talk about his behavior while on the big D. He had no idea he'd been so paranoid, so I explained to him how his liver function wasn't apt to metabolize a medicine as strong as Dilaudid, due to the Hep C. Armed with that knowledge & after leaving me their contact information, we said our goodbyes.

Even though a large number of my patients & their families appreciate the job I do and would like to keep in contact with me, I always walk away feeling as though there was more I should've done.

* * *

My Patient's Husband Pooped on the Floor!

May, 2013

On Sunday I had a 60-something "indigent" female with an ostomy bag. I put indigent in quotes because I myself am currently poor. I've never been poor in my life until recent years, except this is the first time I've had health insurance since 2006.

I liked my patient. She was soft-spoken and ashamed that she won't be able to pay her bill. This I can relate to. Her husband meanwhile, the man with the golden Reeboks, is standing behind me bad-mouthing me. I was warned about him. When he left the room to go on one of his frequent walks, she told me he "hasn't been taking his ADD medicine."

Throughout the day he continued to bad-mouth me, as though he'd snap and sucker punch me, because he was always standing behind me. Once again I find myself terrified in my place of employment. A normal occurrence. Finally I'd had enough of his lip. I asked him what I'd done, and my patient intervened and said, "Nothing! It's his ADD!"

When he left the room again I expressed my concern that this was something more than ADD, & that he ought to visit a Psychiatrist. She told me she couldn't afford mental health care, so I went to look for the social worker. Golden Reeboks returned to the room without acknowledging me in the hall (I swear to you up & down his Reeboks were gold). A few minutes later, that's when I get the call.

"Your patient's husband's choking."

"What??" I ask, while darting into her room.

"Her husband's choking."

And sure enough, he was. He had been eating *her* lunch & was choking on it. I get behind him (this had worked on my mom once before), position myself, and SQUEEZE!!!

I look at him and he's still choking, though now he's making sounds. I run out the room looking for the doctor who'd called me while I was in the process of squeezing the man. I wasn't kidding when I said my phone rings every 3 minutes. The doctor just so happened to be right outside the room. He runs in and also applies the Heimlich to this man. It was then that I realized the horrible smell and what I'd thought was spit-up food on the floor... was actually poop.

We had squeezed the shit out of him.

After one squeeze from me and one squeeze from the doctor, the man was A-OK.

When I walked back into the room later on, the man had fallen asleep on the couch, in his own shit. Smeared all over the floor, all over the couch and into the crevasses too.

Guess who gets to clean this up.

Yep!

The RN with the $75,000 BSN degree and $22/hour job. Mind you, I *often* find myself cleaning up feces, vomit, blood, & piss on this floor. I don't fully understand why the buck is passed (per hospital protocol) from the housekeeper to the RN.

My mental health is in quick decline.

Chapter 2

I've Made an Addict Out of Her

June, 2013

I recently had the pleasure of getting to know a 50-something woman with stomach problems. She would be in the hospital, same room, for over 2 months. That's a big bill.

I didn't like her the second I met her. She was rude, condescending, and made me feel like shit. My LPN had had her the previous summer and told me all about her. I tried to appeal to this woman, I really did.

We had her on a Dilaudid PCA (0.4mg q8min). I know, it's a big dose. And boy would she sit on that thing as soon as it turned green. Rarely would I have to change a patient's PCA cartridge more than once in a shift. But for this woman it was every 4 hours.

She demanded to be bathed even though she was capable of doing it herself.

She could get up and use the bathroom, though she chose to crap in a towel and throw it in the corner (repeatedly).

She didn't like me because I was a straight, white, female... she herself had a white parent with whom she was very close. I cannot comprehend the racial bias, and I consider myself lucky for this. My LPN was not straight, so she adored her.

She came from another part of the country & let's just say that her personality had not adjusted, nor would it ever.

Imagine having Kim Kardashian as a patient. Forced to stay in a ghetto hospital for 2 months, with a hospital room just the same as everybody else on the floor. This woman truly thought she was God.

She'd have rich friends come by to visit, bring her huge amounts of fancy foods, and as soon as they'd leave she'd throw up. I told her it was because of the pain medicine. She was my patient on 5 different occasions and she was constantly under the influence of the same amount of Dilaudid as the week before. Nothing had changed.

She had a picc in her arm but got a thrombus so we had to switch sides, just so she could continue to pump the Big D into her vein. Then she got a thrombus in the other arm, but she fought so hard against removing it (because she wanted to remain high - I know this, I'm not stupid). I have no idea why she was in the hospital, aside for some abdominal pain. Nor after 2 months had they solved anything just short of sending her home with a brand new drug habit.

As her nurse this naturally worried me. I didn't want her to resort to buying contraband off the street to slam, since she'd never been a drug abuser before. After bad-mouthing all of the doctors, their opinions of her fell even lower, and eventually she was cut loose.

I feel it was against my morals to be treating her drug habit. I wasn't doing my job or taking care of her medical needs. There was no improvement in 2 months. The Charge Nurse told me she was a manipulative bitch who was wasting a room on the floor. The team of doctors agreed.

This was a high-maintenance waste of time and eventually, none of us cared anymore.

* * *

Dragonbreath Psych Patient & My First Med Error

June, 2013

I've never had my very own psych patient outside of nursing school. I mean a true psych patient, diagnosis and behavior. Well today I had my first.

50-something woman with spinal surgery, J collar, schizophrenia, smelly butt crack. And the worst breath I'd ever smelled in my life. Remember, I must often bend down close to her to change her position & help her pee, 'cause she can't move herself too well. She has refused to continue receiving IV medication, including her pain meds.

But she wants her p.o. Valium and she wants it NOW.

In the first place, I'd been a nervous wreck since this morning because I wasn't sure *"what would happen on this day,"* what with having a pretty vulgar psych patient & such. My favorite LPN, the one who's a lesbian, knows this woman. She teaches me that "Dragonbreath" is appeased with coffee.

In nursing school they taught us to never "make deals" with this type of patient. As a real nurse in the field with serious time constraints however? You're forced to.

But this didn't work for very long anyway.

18

I forgot to mention that she has a sitter: one of our precious 2 PCT's. *All day.* So when the PCT has to go for her 30-45 minute lunch, guess who has to sit with Dragonbreath.

Me.

I didn't get to eat lunch that day... again (this is part of a nurse's life and I've grown to accept it).

Now, feeling as though I was neglecting my other patients, I hurry to the med room & pull out a 5mg Valium. I rush to give it to her, and all is well for the next 2 hours. Then another LPN comes to me and asks why I removed a Valium from her patient's name.

Oh shit!

I could feel my license slipping away.

Again.

Apparently, her patient had the same last name as mine, & in my haste I did not notice the first names were different. So I call the doctor and tell her what happened. She asked how Dragonbreath was & I said she was A-OK. She laughed and said just to make an incident report, & that it was no big deal. I told the Charge Nurse & did just that.

At this point I became very discouraged. That other LPN gave me a tight hug and told me not to worry myself to death, and that it had happened to her when she was younger. That I should be relieved that it wasn't a dangerous drug.

But I wasn't relieved. Not one bit. As a matter of fact I had been so damn uneasy & on-edge ever since I set foot on this floor, for reasons such as this! I felt incompetent and undeserving of the title of RN, no matter how meager the pay was.

I was mad at myself, but I got over it.

Over the course of the following week I never had Dragonbreath again, but I could hear her screaming from her bed while I was in the hallway.

This time I *was* relieved.

* * *

Discharge Me IMMEDIATELY!!!

July, 2013

Have I mentioned before how poorly managed this floor is?

Well today I get to work and there is a patient who does not have a nurse assigned to her.

You heard me right.

So guess who gets stuck with this bitch. And only because I noticed her in the hallway, pacing, and I made the mistake of asking her nicely, "Can I help you?"

This witch started demanding I discharge her by 9 am, not a second later. Why? Because she wants to go to her baby girl's beauty pageant the following day. This woman is a white trash bitch and you can tell a mile away.

My patient in the next room has been suffering a stroke since night shift went off duty. Her doctor is this patient's doctor also. He can't leave this patient's side and I explain to her why not.

She doesn't care!

She goes to the middle of the floor, the atrium, the center of everything, and starts bitching to me and the Charge Nurse in front of all the visitors and doctors. I was so embarrassed.

Things like this, I've been informed by other nurses who've worked here for decades, have been occurring on a daily basis at this hospital, ever since the hurricane several years back. It's begun to make the hospital look like a trashy place to most of the self-respecting patients and their families.

And why? Because the hospital had begun to take on a lower class of patient. Criminals & the like. The flood gates were open, truthfully, and they are taking in EVERY kind of patient, no filter. This was when it was made certain to me that this hospital has lost its reputation, and is no longer worth dealing with, whether as an employer or a provider.

I say this because this type of patient has no intention of paying their bill, and yes that does matter because medical staff aren't slaves. We have student loans! And then the patients who do pay their bills get stuck with rising costs to make up for this lost revenue.

Certain things in life I make sure to avoid: going to Walmart on a Friday night, passing through the projects, certain interstate entrances...

Many doctors & nurses can do it, but I cannot. I grew up in this city but I moved out of it for a reason. Perhaps now it's time to search for employment in a more rural place.

Needless to say, I had her out of there by 9:30 am.

* * *

You Ain't Nothin' but a Hound Dog

July, 2013

You know who they are the instant they hit the floor: "Ohhh Jee-zuss!" The severe, uncontrolled pain. It happens to all of us and on some floors, like this one, it happens every single day.

You instantly know that you won't be seeing your other patients for the next hour, while trying to contact a doctor to get this woman some adequate pain relief. On top of admitting and fully assessing her, you see that she's already been given something on the previous floor.

Well it ain't workin'.

I spend a lot of time getting to know my patients. Socializing keeps depression away, at least for me. I like the feeling that my patients are comfortable confiding in me, all of them so far.

So this lady tells me that she takes a lot of narcotic pain medicine to combat the pain from a degenerated knee joint. She's a 50-something waitress in relatively good shape, but I already know that by taking narcotic pain meds daily, she's gonna have a high tolerance.

This is a teaching hospital. The interns are so very swamped in such a hectic environment, I always wonder how it is that they keep their cool. They never really look or sound stressed out, even when they've gone 2 days without a wink (or a shower). I don't know how they do it.

Uncontrolled pain is a situation I do not like, and have had to deal with far too many times on the post-op floor. But I think I've started learning how to combat it. With the dosage increase, my new patient got the relief she needed, and my stress & contemplation from earlier had been all for nothing.

Unlike my other uncontrolled pain patients, she didn't throw a fit, so I could rest easy.

Now, what will *tomorrow* bring?

Chapter 3

The Husband Complains because it's Too Hot

August, 2013

I want to talk about chronic pain and high-acuity.

Here is an example of a patient that is high-acuity, and the type this floor is always serving:

30-something female in the hospital for hip replacement. This is her 6th hip replacement in 4 years. She had gotten into a car accident when she was 15 years old, and as a result has left foot drop which will never go away, and severe life-long pain on top of that.

She is on a plethora of narcotics:

6 po MS Contin (I forget the dose) q12h

1 mg Xanax q8h

1.5 mg Dilaudid IV q2h prn

5 po Hydrocodone (? dose) q4h prn

1-2 Oxycontin q12h (? dose)

My heart goes out to her as when I come on shift, she is crying and in pain. I spent the whole day with the doctors trying to figure out a way to improve her pain. We added something else to the mix, I forget what, but you get my drift.

This time it worked!

I had heard about it before, but this was the first experience I had with a patient setting an alarm in her iPhone for each of her scheduled doses. I am not even trying to joke.

But for what it's worth, I know she's not a "seeker." This is just her daily regimen & something she has to live with.

I have to get her up myself to the toilet several times a day. I mean, her dear hubby points to the commode and says, "Empty it!"

I have to keep my tested tongue in my mouth.

Where is the PCT, you ask?

That's a great question!

I also have to help the physical therapist get her up & ambulate. I am in her room when her pain comes back, as it does every few hours, giving her a back rub and talking to her. She does not ever want me to leave her room and because she needs constant tending-to, I hardly do leave. It's either that or she calls me every few minutes. Thank God my other two patients are low maintenance.

Her husband is always there.

I have this lady for three days straight and as the days go by, he becomes more and more of an asshole. At first it's a thousand-watt smile as he turns on the charm. But then he begins to complain that it's too hot in the room. Which it is, because the a/c units in this hospital are not up to par and are probably from the 1960's.

But he is not my patient. My patient is comfortable in her room and that is what matters to me.

When I do get a minute to go check on my other patients, he goes to the desk repeatedly demanding a different room. This halts everything for me, because then the secretary calls me.

What the fuck am I supposed to do about it? I have people's damn health to take care of. This is dangerous!

On the 3rd day of our brief sisterhood, she has asked her husband to leave. Then she tells me what a dick he truly is and that she wants to get a divorce. She says that all he does at home is stand out in his man cave and smoke cigarettes. He won't even take his cancer-ridden dog to the vet! The poor animal.

Although I felt as though I had made a new friend, I was completely drained by the end of my shift. I was drained in a way that I had never felt before. I'm sure she was appreciative of me, as she gave me a very genuine hug when I went off shift (2 hours late, even though I had an hour's drive ahead of me).

I had spoken several times to the Nurse Supervisor about instating visitor hours for this very reason. When did visitor hours go out of style? This makes it very hard for nurses to do their jobs, because these people get in our way. I figured, if we complained loud enough then something would get done.

Boy was I wrong.

Like I always say, "Happy nurses = happy patients = great Press-Ganey scores."

This hospital now has a terrible patient satisfaction score, and yet they keep buying every single other hospital in the region. I don't understand this.

* * *

Show Me Your Culo?

August, 2013

One of the good things that has come out of this nightmare are the relationships I form with my patients. Sometimes it's not such a good thing.

My 20-something female patient from The Sticks is in with "constipation" & abdominal pain. This woman's super obese. She has 4 sets of breasts and I'll tell you how I know: the floor I work on gets so damn hot in the summer time. I call the maintenance men every single day and they fix the a/c, but the next day it seems to be out again. Yes, this is in the U.S.

And so my patient is stark naked *all day long* in her room. Her husband & mom are by her side without fail. When her mom's out of the room, my patient informs me that she & her husband are swingers and they have a crush on my lesbian LPN. But I tell them to please not bother her about such things, as she was going through a personal tragedy & wouldn't be in the mood.

Oh yeah. This is a weird couple.

Well several months later, I see her mom in the hallway. We say hi and I ask what's wrong. She tells me the girl has had to have spinal surgery.

While waiting for the elevator with another nurse, I see the girl roll up to me in a wheelchair. The other nurse was a very polite lady. The girl pulls out her iPhone & shows me a picture of her asshole. With a brown spot next to it.

I gotta get out of this place. I gotta leave here.

The other nurse gets a weird look on her face, and me? I act like it's completely normal to assess assholes from the hallway. I told the girl I had no idea what it could be, and to inform her doctor of it... and that I really was pressed for time.

I think this was the only day in months that I actually got to go downstairs to buy lunch. Never mind that I had just finished looking at the photo of an anus. Dammit I was hungry!

Even with the strangeness of this woman, I kinda felt happy to see her again. A friendly face in a miserable place, I guess.

* * *

Stop Everything! Blitzed Out Hall-Walker Wants Ranch Dressing!

September, 2013

I love being kind to visitors and patients who aren't mine. After all, it's an enormous hospital and people get lost. I enjoy the same kind of courtesy.

Another impossibly busy day and I'm coming out of my patient's room, on the way to another patient and I'm in quite a hurry. This is not the time for me to be stopped by anyone, as I need my concentration unbroken.

Too bad, because I run smack into a creepy young blonde wearing a camouflage shirt. Her hair's stringy and you could tell she was high as a kite. Probably Dilaudid. She looks like the type who tells you she's "allergic to Morphine, Hydrocodone..." and throws a fit if the doctor won't prescribe Dilaudid for her.

Well she's looking at me like she's about to make a time-consuming request. You know the look.

"Can I help you?" I ask her.

"I need some Ranch dressing. You got any?"

So now I have to walk so damn far away to sift through the bag in the fridge and see if there is any Ranch. There is none.

I go back and tell her this, and then I turn and try to remember what important health concern I was on my way to address in the first place.

Several hours later I get taken aside and "talked to." This bitch complained that I wouldn't bring her any Ranch dressing. My Charge Nurse knows there isn't any and so this is all futile. I told her I was polite to the broad, and the Charge Nurse nods her head and says she knows already, and not to worry about it.

So why take me aside in the first place? Why honor these brats & junkies? Who in the Hell has time to deal with this shit?

Not me, that's for sure.

* * *

Semi-Private Rooms & HIPAA (& You!)

September, 2013

Let's talk about semi-private rooms.

In this hospital they're the size of my closet and there are 2 hospital beds crammed into each one of them. They're always full too. There's a small table & a "privacy curtain" in between them. Each patient pays $1,000 a night for one of these beds. There is no room for their visitors but someone always insists we squeeze a recliner in there (times two). There are scratches & holes all over the walls from decades of equipment being moved and nurses having to squeeze in there too.

I hate semi-private rooms. I hate 'em with a passion.

Not only because it's impossible to get to bed B when another nurse is at bed A, but it's always a HIPAA violation waiting to happen. Once again, our licenses are on the line.

Quite often the patient in bed A wants to know how the patient in bed B is doing. I've gotten used to telling these polite inquirers that I'm not allowed to share that information, in the name of HIPAA. Never mind that the patient in bed B is hard of hearing, so the doctor and I have had to shout all of his confidential information at him already as it is. The patient in bed A is now aware of everything.

I sometimes hear about the code that took place shortly before I came on board. The reason it's become a legend is because of how horribly it went down. We have codes every week on this floor, but only 3 or 4 patients die per year. At this point I still haven't realized how bad of a statistic this is.

The legend goes as follows:

The patient in bed B has coded and the usual responders show up (every single nurse on the floor, 5 interns, 2 residents, several patient visitors, and the floor supervisor). Nothing is being done and nobody who knows what to do can gain access to bed B, because the rooms are so cramped as it is. So the floor supervisor must climb over the patient in bed A in order to reach the coding patient in bed B.

They perform their heroic measures but to no avail. The patient has died.

Now the body must be transferred out of the room and down to the morgue. How to do this in a semi-private room? They fold the bed with the body still in it, squeeze it through between the wall & bed A, and direct it out the door. The patient in bed A is completely mortified.

Just as I am. At myself. For not quitting when I had the chance.

Hospitals started out as public wards. There weren't even any privacy curtains in between the beds. This was in the days when mankind was actually grateful & moral.

But because of cross-contamination concerns & better quality of care when a patient's privacy is honored, wards were divided up into semi-private rooms.

Now in the days of entitlement and HIPAA, private rooms are all the rage. And I like them so much more because they're easy to move around in.

HIPAA came to be in the early 2000's. You would think by now hospitals will have updated in order to accommodate this very important set of laws. But they haven't. There are so many semi-private rooms on this floor.

They see this as more beds = more patients = more money. And this is all they care about. It is completely up to the doctors and nurses, as always, to make extra time and find extra ways in which to prevent their licenses from being revoked (*for some reason or another*).

I guess the best way to describe how we as nurses feel on this floor is this: ***SITTING DUCKS!***

Chapter 4

The Only Drug That Works for Me Starts With a "D"...

October, 2013

I often think about the concept of not judging my patients, and being as compassionate as any human can be. I realize most patients are uncomfortable, nervous, & often in pain. I never hesitate, after careful evaluation, to shoot up a patient per request... even when I know it's not truthfully needed. I'm just not gonna stand there & argue with them about something so subjective.

So how does one know if a person isn't really in pain? I don't mean mild cramps and soreness. I mean the full-blown, top of the chart pain. It goes a little something like this:

I walk into room.

Young, petite female is sitting on commode taking a dump. Father is directly across from her.

"What's your level of pa..."

"A TEN!" She smiles at me.

I bend down to perform the push.

>>poot!craaap!stiiink!<<

I keep a straight face.

"I like your hair," she spouts with a smile. Mind you, I've only pushed half a millimeter so far.

It goes on like this all day, every two-and-a-half hours. This is obviously time-consuming, but there is nothing we can do but comply & vent in the lunch room.

And what would a good argument be against emptying out a patient's Pyxis drawer per request, so long as it's ordered? I sensibly adhere to this.

Here's another example:

Frequent flyer, 20-something female "cancer survivor" and many, many other things. She's passed to me because my LPN doesn't want to deal with her (again). The first time I ever saw her, she was being "guided" down the hall by the PCT to her new private room. There were two other nurses with me and as soon as she saw us, the act began: walking slow and painfully, taking careful steps... "Aye. Aye. Aye." I mean this is how I used to act as a child, when I wanted to stay home from school.

I go into the room to talk & get to know her. After setting her up with a delicious Dilaudid & Ativan cocktail, we get to talking some more. I clean & replace her JP dressing, and then leave the room. She turned out to be a pretty cool person.

Except that she's a substance abuser.

Ain't no matter what substance, she'll take it all. My LPN grew to despise her so badly, she looked her up on Facebook. Photo after photo of her in glamorous outfits, getting ready to party out on the town. In one hand a daiquiri, in the other a joint.

I'm back in her room later on in the day and I realize she has applied eye-liner. I was jealous at how *perfectly* she'd gotten it on. Then her sisters were visiting with her, in from smoking cigarettes (I guess). She became so comfortable with me as her nurse, she decided to drop the act. See, she knew I was gonna show up on the spot and deliver her legal high. And I feel that if she had in fact had cancer previously, it's possible she picked up the addiction while under treatment.

These are the ethical dilemma. Yes I judged her, so what? If we don't deliver these legal highs fashionably & on time, we will get a complaint & *negative patient satisfaction scores!!!*

And why should it be such a moral problem in my mind? Giving someone a legal high is making them feel good, right? It's appeasing them. I like making people feel good.

But I still can't shake the feeling that it's morally wrong to aid in a person's sinking further into dependence.

Often I think that a lot of today's adults are very much like children, and they seem to have fewer and fewer morals.

* * *

Drinking Coffee All Day

October, 2013

Today I was teamed up with an LPN from my neck of the woods. Same upbringing, same ghetto attitude if need be. And I stress the "if need be" part for myself only. This lady isn't afraid to show her displeasure, whereas I am.

Our patient is a 50-something from another part of the city. Her whole family is in the room, including her wheelchair-bound daddy. It was this type of patient: 1 mg IV Dilaudid q3h prn. Like I've told you before, I'm Johnny on the Spot with pain relief.

She has an odd-looking IV in her left AC, which I notice early on is showing signs of pending infiltration (a tad leaky, harder & harder to push). I don't know what kind of IV it is, so I call anesthesia and describe it to them. "That's a rapid-infusion IV. You can take it out if you want to."

The only problem is that in this hospital, RN's aren't allowed to remove picc lines. And this type of IV removal or tampering has never been considered by the lawmakers. So even the Charge Nurse doesn't know if I should remove it or not.

Because it could become a problem with infection, my subconscious is telling me to pull the damn thing out. But in the end, I just decide to leave it. Another example of "trouble with my license" should one of the lawmakers find out about this and object to it.

I've heard horror stories about this hospital throwing its nurses under the bus and reporting them to the BON to keep the hospital safe from prosecution. This is another tidbit that fuels my fears on a daily basis.

Anyway. She's not getting all the Dilaudid she wants and she's crying about it. I put an IV in her right arm but before doing so, I'm having trouble finding a vein. Hers are all shriveled.

The LPN comes in to give it a try and the woman says, "Do y'all know what you're doing?" in a very rude manner. I had spent some time with this woman in the morning and so far I had gotten along well with her. But I hate people who have no manners, especially when they're old enough to have picked up some common decency.

In the meantime I start to have problems with another patient, and they require my full attention. When I go back into this woman's room she is visibly pissed and on her cell phone. "I've been calling y'all for the past hour. Where were you!!!"

To which daddy answers, "They just stand around all day drinking coffee in the hall!"

And then her mother answers, "Don't be so rude! What's wrong with y'all?" I like her elderly mother.

While she is on the cell phone, she sees that I have brought her shot of Dilaudid. Does she put the phone down? No. No she does not. This is a woman in her 50's.

Finally my LPN can take it no longer. "Ma'am can you please put the phone down so she can give you the shot?" to which the woman complies.

I'm having to learn the hard way how to be an assertive person.

It was an OK day, despite the aggravation. And what her dad said had me boiling with anger. Why do patients and visitors feel this way? The only nurse he could have seen "standing around drinking coffee" was an older nurse who has two different jobs and is trying to stay awake.

What's wrong with these people?

* * *

Why I Became a Nurse

November, 2013

When I was in the 2nd grade I knew I wanted to be a nurse. My beloved grandmother had turned me onto the legend that was Florence Nightingale, and the following year I dressed up as her on History Day.

As a freshman in high school I started volunteering at the local hospital, and did so until I was 17. My love for medicine and patient care grew substantially.

I went to an all girls' Catholic high school. Feminism was still a popular idea in the 90's, though now I can see the damage it has done. We were taught that we should "aim high" and we "could do whatever we put our minds to." This is an ideal I normally embrace. But lately I have a problem with instilling unrealistic expectations into the minds of the young.

At my high school, they didn't bring in nurses, paralegals, secretaries, home makers, flight attendants, teachers, or even lawyers or pilots. No, they brought in a brain surgeon, a rocket scientist, and a judge. I kid you not. Those of us who would go on to become these things (3 girls in a class of 116), didn't need this kind of encouragement. They were gonna do it anyway.

So the voice in my head repeated the mantra of these uber-successful women, and constantly told me to "aim higher!" So instead of nursing school, I went into pre-med. I wanted to be like the neurosurgeon lady who'd come and talked to us. She

42

was so smart and accomplished. Never mind that I already knew I sucked at Chemistry & Physics, two subjects requiring at least a B in order to gain admission to an American medical school. No... never mind that. I was gonna do it!

Since my Chemistry & Physics grades also sucked in college, I applied and got accepted to a medical school in Germany. Yeah, I know. So I learned German and went. We had to take a German proficiency course prior to starting our field of study, and when I passed that, they informed me that there were no more places left, and that I'd have to register under another major until a seat freed up for me.

Devastation is not the word. And this is the problem with universities in the predominantly socialist countries: completely filled up with lifelong students. After being there for two years and still no seat, I decided I wanted to come home.

Because I couldn't afford nursing school upon returning, I would have to work odd jobs for the next 7 years. And even then, I had only saved up enough to afford the first 2 years of nursing school. After that, I had to take out a loan.

But I did it. Even while losing my grandmother to CHF, I made it through.

My first year of nursing turned out to be an utter nightmare for me, but I haven't given up. I won't give up either because this is a job that I generally enjoy being at. I write mostly about my bad experiences because I feel this is a great outlet and a nice way to share things with other people.

I like to tuck people in, change their dressings, give them medicines, and see them get better. Even the ones who are dying, I like to comfort them & make them laugh. I mean, I live for this shit. I guess it brings me closer to my grandma in many ways.

I like the social aspect of nursing: I'm constantly meeting new members of the community, and I keep in touch with a good deal of them. I like working with doctors and learning from them a lot about physiology.

This was what I was supposed to have done a long time ago. I can't help but regret losing 13 years of work experience as a nurse, and part of me wants to place blame on what we were told in high school.

Were we set up for failure and disappointment? Because most of us did go on to fail, and have had to get up and try again (& again). Some girls did not get up. Either way, the blame always comes back to me, myself, & I.

I guess if I ever have children, I'll know to teach them to do what they feel they wanna do, and not "what would be *even better*." This just goes against the fates and nature. A person can really go far when starting at a low-paying but enjoyable place. Just stick with it & climb the ladder, that's the key. This is how experts are made.

* * *

El Dia de los Culos, or: Code Brown

November, 2013

Today is Sunday. You know what Sunday is?

It's game day, that's what.

On my 49 bed floor (soon-to-be 53!), the hospital agrees to hire two (2) and only two PCTs. Keep in mind this is an inner city post-operative floor. No specialties. Anything operated on and it comes here. Also any overflow, drug detox, suicide watch, psych emergencies, observations, etc. Not what any of us were told upon applying nor during the interview. This however poses an awful lot of valuable skills for the new nurse to pick up.

Yeah, yeah, yeah.

With it being football day, both PCT's call out sick, as do 4 nurses. They're all sick. All of 'em.

Sick.

Our max number of patients is 5 per nurse. This might seem like a good deal, but one quickly learns what high acuity really means, even when working with 3 such patients. There is no comparison. I'd rather have 6 low acuity patients than 3 high ones.

Today I have 4 high-acuity patients, 2 of them are out of their minds and all of them are bowel incontinent. And we have no PCT's today.

One of my patients comes to me from The Sticks. He was climbing a tree on the hunt for grub worms (for bait), when he cascaded down & broke his pelvis. Ouch! He's an older, overweight man, and today he has terrible diarrhea. Is it ever fantastic?

I'm in his room cleaning him up when I hear the intercom in the next room, and that patient's private PCT requesting my assistance. That patient was also in need of another cleaning. I don't like for my patients to lie in their own mess, so I hurried next door.

Upon returning to the med room so I could pass my 9 am meds (at 11 am), the secretary stops me & tells me that my patient from The Sticks' daughter, who's an LPN, came to complain about me (ME) for her daddy's transport folder being "carelessly" left in his room. Mind you, transport left the folder there. Transport = high school boys. Not that I even had a split second to inspect this man's room, as he was constantly in a bad mood and needed tending to.

But no, I fucked up. Again.

What do these people expect from one person? What this woman was doing was implying that I myself left the folder there, and was too lazy and unconcerned to be bothered by it. I'd spent literally all morning cleaning up the multiple accidents of 4 people. Not what I went to nursing school for. Not what I went into $75,000 worth of debt for. And it's not a rare occurrence. I'm always, every day cleaning up shit!

I'm beginning to really hate this place. Maybe I hated it from day one and am only just now able to admit it. If it keeps up like this, I'll be looking for a new place of employment.

Chapter 5

The Manipulative Poly-substance Abuser

December, 2013

Today was another bad day, but it wasn't terrible.

I had a 40-something male patient who had coaxed local cops into a high-speed, liquor-induced motorcycle chase and he crashed. His right leg was terribly broken and he was now in an immobilizer until he could have surgery. The thing was smelly and infected.

He had a chubby female friend constantly by his side, rolling him around the hospital in a wheelchair. Every hour he'd go out to smoke. And he's an extremely loud person.

I go in to meet and assess him, and he decides he likes me right away. He continues to complain about how he's now got a lawyer to sue the crap out of the police department. My brother is a lawyer and he talks about it sometimes. In my heart I knew that this guy had no case, yet there was still a desperate lawyer out there who was willing to take it.

The police had asked him to stop the motorcycle because he was clearly intoxicated and he was speeding. Thus ensued a high-speed chase. I mean in excess of 100 mph, during which the cops went after him, warned him that they would hit him with their SUV if he didn't stop, and followed through with their promise.

Because of course he didn't stop. No siree. The rules do not apply to him.

So now he's convinced that pretty soon, he'll be a millionaire.

When the friend rolls him in the halls he is very obnoxious. The other nurses & visitors know to stay as far away from him as possible. It's just something in the natural instincts. "Stay away from a person like this. Just avoid it altogether."

My Charge Nurse told me this was "anti-social" behavior, and though I know by now he's not a nut job, he's still not a desirable patient. That, and his wounded leg stinks.

I see in his chart that he's got a history as a poly-substance abuser. So the doctor only prescribes 2mg IV Dilaudid q12h. I thought this was a bit conservative, but he wasn't writhing in pain. And by talking to him I learn that he lives on friends' couches. He's also an insomniac and he changes his damn dressing every hour, on the hour, "to keep it clean."

But he seems to be having a good ol' time in the hospital.

Finally the doctor orders a PCA for him, so I hook it up. While I'm doing so, he begins to ask me what would it take to open the cartridge & get to the Dilaudid. I tell him he'd be in trouble & I'd be in trouble and to please just follow the rules (for once). Then he tells me he's going to throw the pump down in an attempt to break it, extract the Dilaudid, & replace it with Saline. I explain the concept of overdose & death, and once again, I plead with him not to do this.

In the meantime I notice something out the corner of my eye. When I look down, I see that it's the fattest cockroach I'd ever seen in my life! I start to freak out because I have some kind of phobia towards roaches. Sure, this is a run-down floor. But dammit, we never had a roach problem. I'm thinking it got into his female friend's bag before she came to the hospital. These people are dirty. It's not a surprise.

After the roach is murdered by a male nurse, I go to my computer to chart & make a long note about the conversation we just had. If he should happen to follow through with his plan, then I don't want to get in trouble. I decided that making a note wasn't good enough, so I tell the Charge Nurse just to cover my ass.

Then I get a frantic call from him. He wants to see his nurse.

I go in there and he's livid. He tells me that he had finally managed to fall asleep as the dietary man burst into his room with his food... and that he'd like to file a complaint. On this floor there is no patient advocate. The nurse is to play this role and fulfill a patient's every waking request. And because I'd never done this before, I go to the Charge Nurse to see what can be done.

The answer is nothing. Nothing can be done. There are no complaint forms for him to fill out. It takes me 30 minutes to tend to this issue, because the Nurse Supervisor was off the floor and nobody knew what to do. So in the end, no complaint was filed and he had fallen asleep again anyway.

Once again, I got yanked around and lost precious time.

I told the Charge Nurse I would not be wanting him back the next day, and she honored my request.

* * *

Party in the Parking Lot

December, 2013

I don't understand what it is about inner-city hospitals, but the habitants of The Sticks and Ghetto seem to think this is a vacation resort.

And why wouldn't they? There are 3 restaurants, a hair & nail salon, and countless shops on the bottom floor.

I'm driving through the parking lot on my way in to work (at 11 am), and there's a rowdy bunch, I mean a *whole* bunch of people who look like they're on their way up to visit a patient. They're all carrying beer. Beer? Seriously, at 11 am? I almost freak out, and all this before I even got inside. This is getting too crazy & it's turning me into an old, grumpy bitch really fast.

These are the visitors (during the day) who cram themselves into a semiprivate room with no regard for the other patient who's trying to sleep. They reek of smoke & booze, are foul-mouthed and have rotten attitudes. They lack manners and get in my way when I need to take care of the patient.

I've expressed my concern about visitors to my boss. I'm not the only one who has a problem with the non-existent visiting hours. Every single day-shift nurse has complained.

These people get the run of the floor and they make me lose time fulfilling their requests. If I don't fulfill their requests, they'll coax the patient into leaving a bad satisfaction card. Couldn't have that now could we? Even though there are signs that say, "Shhh patients resting!" they still let their children run up and down, screaming & wailing.

And nobody bats an eyelash at this, except the nurses.

I think it's important for nurse bosses and hospital administrators to remember this key fact: happy nurses = happy patients = more $$$ for the hospital.

Maybe it's time I consider switching to night shift.

* * *

One Big Clusterfuck

January, 2014

I was reading a friend's post on Facebook the other day. She declared it was discharge time at the hospital and she was feelin' much better. Of course her friends and family soon started flooding the comment section asking questions like, "What happened? Are you alright?"

Apparently neither she nor her treatment team knew what the cause of her temporary ailing was. And then I read something that pissed me off.

One of the female elders in her family writes down, "You better not leave that hospital!!! DEMAND to know what was wrong with you!!!"

Oh that's good.

Does the public think the medical staff is holding out on them just for shits & giggles?

The answer is no, no they're not. The public needs to learn the meaning of the term "idiopathic."

The problem with many people today is we all feel we're entitled, and that we're deserving of priority and the royal treatment. The trouble is, none of us is royalty anymore and we gotta stand in line and wait like everybody else, unless we've got some extra money on hand, then by all means... to the front of the line.

Which reminds me of another thing about my floor that bothers me and yet at the same time I somewhat agree with: V.I.P. status. If you can pay the extra money, then why not?

These folks (they're always nice and never a problem) come onto an already full house, and they're put on the top of the list for a private room, bypassing everybody. I imagine this entails paying an extra hefty price, but they have the means to do so. On the chart there's even a label right by their code status, and it reads "VIP." And we know what this means.

We don't get extra pay. No, we won't see a single red cent of that extra money they'll be paying. But administration does, most certainly!

There's more of a silent rule that if we don't drop everything at once and answer their calls immediately, there'll be hell to pay. They always give me the V.I.P.'s because I'm soft-spoken, friendly, and well-mannered.

One morning my wealthy patient was requesting Dilaudid and I had just come on shift. Her husband wasn't too thrilled with the night shift (he was on the Board of Directors), so he called the Head Nurse and complained. Within two minutes my Charge Nurse was riding my ass. This happened yet again until I was able to get my ducks in a row. The doctor even called me to tell me I could give her as much

Dilaudid as she wanted, prior to her surgery (yes, we also take pre-ops... I told you, we take everything).

I ended up bonding with this couple, and the husband even called his Board to put in a compliment for me. I told him he didn't need to do that. I could sense lately that I wouldn't be working here for very much longer. I didn't like... no, I HATED the way the nurses were treated and beaten down like rented mules... and never compensated for it.

I mean, doctors and nurses are what make a hospital's existence possible. Along with the respiratory techs, radiology, pharmacy, the cleaning ladies, etc. Not administration. At this hospital there are so many more administrative positions as there are medical staff.

Don't get me wrong. I do understand the need for basic administrative duties, marketing, finance, etc. But I invite you to check out some of the administrative titles in job postings. Only look in the career sections of large & enormous hospitals, then you'll see what I'm talking about. And I guarantee these people are paid more. And yes, it matters!

Because when this happens, a hospital turns to shit. It happens every time!

We had a deep freeze recently and many nurses couldn't make it that way (when this happens in the South, everything shuts down completely). The nurses who did have to spend several days and nights at the hospital were promised handsome compensation, but not in writing. There was no time for that. When the hospital did not follow through with this promise, all hell broke loose. This issue was never resolved. It was swept under the rug because after all, we nurses are mere $22/hour peons.

Several of the nurses quit, as expected; but several more new grads were hired immediately at the cost of $30,000 each in orientation fees. I believe the brunt of this money goes to pay for the speech the CEO gives at the enormous "Welcome New Hires!" ceremony.

I feel very sorry for them.

PS: The CEO is a man from very far away who doesn't even have a background in medicine. Somehow he knew the right person and landed this job. That's how things work in this city. He's a sweet man and very qualified to work in a high-paying job, but CEO of a major hospital? C'mon!!!

* * *

My Patient Has Left the Building

January, 2014

One of our Charge Nurses recently had a patient exit the floor. That's right, our Charge Nurses even have to take on patients due to the sheer amount we get.

This was a psych patient. Surprise, surprise! And a suicide threat. So why did they assign this patient to the room right next to the elevator? Why?

This is nowhere near the nurses' station. And of course this nurse was busy with another patient at the other end of the hospital (they always assign like this, that's one reason I've lost so much weight. Another is because I never eat lunch. No time to do so). And so her patient just ups and leaves.

She gets into a little bit of trouble because she is a "pet," never mind pinpointing where exactly the problem lay: in accepting beyond capacity so much so that they will resort to stuffing a flight risk right by the elevators. This is desperation, desperation for more patient capacity and more nurses to evenly distribute the brunt. But this hospital will never admit to this desperation, and in turn faces hundreds of lawsuits and millions of dollars' worth of lost income per year. But Admin still gets their bonus every year. I bet just the bonus of one of these people would be enough to pay off my student loan debt.

A few days after this I also receive an attempted suicide/flight risk patient. They put him in an adequate room, but he doesn't want to stay. Now I have to have security on stand-by because this boy is my prisoner. While I'm taking care of my other patients I'm constantly worrying that I'll go into his room & he'll be gone.

My license is endangered.

Meanwhile I get a stab victim, a big muscular man who looks like he became a bodybuilder while in prison. He and his girlfriend are funny and nice, but he's terribly hungry, and can he leave to go get some food? No, I tell him, please don't, because then I'll get in trouble. Although he was perfectly fine to do so in my opinion, it was still against policy.

I go into his room later on and he's gone. For an hour. I'm panicking and about to lose my mind when my phone rings, "Your patient just shit himself."

Oh my God!

I have to go tell the charge nurse that my patient has gone AWOL, and of course take care of my other patients. When I go into my messed patient's room I find the secretary's cleaning his shit up. The secretary. Thank God for her! Now I can tend to my issue. Luckily the other patient returned with a big bag of food. I was off the hook!

How odd is it that we're stretched so damn thin, that the secretary has to help out? I've never seen or heard of this on any functional hospital floor. Once again I confirm that this is a terribly managed, toxic place and the kind of stress we endure is so not worth the daily two-hour commute and the measly paycheck!

There *is* the team-work.

But how did I get myself into this mess?

Chapter 6

A Nurse Who Stays Glued to Her Phone

February, 2014

On our floor the concept of teamwork is always in full-force. Often we are so understaffed we have to have a nurse from another floor float on ours. I think this is pretty common in most hospitals. Regardless of this, you hardly ever see a nurse spending time on her cell phone or piddling around.

Then there's this one nurse who I noticed a long time ago.

I don't like her. She doesn't speak one word to any of the nurses on our floor. She passes her meds, sits down to chart, and then sits on her iPhone. It is inexcusable in our minds to leave a nurse who needs help hanging, yet this kid does it every time she's on our floor.

When the nurse in need goes around asking for help, she sits there deaf & mute, as though she is invisible. Maybe she is deaf; I mean she always has her headphones on... another floor no-no. Yet I've noticed she is one of the "pets" of the new Nurse Supervisor (our former supervisor, the bitch, was only on this floor for a year. Should tell you something).

Good nurses are fired pretty often from this hospital, yet incompetents like this one are loved by the higher ups... all because they are friends or relatives of the people in charge. Everybody complains about this, and yet again, nothing is done.

I have recently applied to a different hospital, one that is much closer to my house and has a better reputation.

* * *

Trouble with the BON, or: My Life is Over

March 15, 2014 - May, 2015

So finally it happened. What I'd been afraid of all along.

My dad had gone into the hospital in January due to a bad pneumonia. He hadn't improved and last month he had to be operated on. There was a large empyema on his left posterior lung lobe, and the operation was four hours long. Followed by a week-long stay in the ICU, with some incidents. This whole time he was under sedation and ventilation (& a chest tube). We didn't know if he was going to make it. I am very, very close to my dad.

At the exact same time, my cousin goes home to find my uncle on the floor, unresponsive. He is taken to the hospital and suffers a heart attack & kidney failure (all at once). On top of that, he learns he will have to have a double BKA, due to diabetic neuropathy leading to distal toe necrosis. I am also close to my uncle.

And at the same time, I am packing up all my stuff because I will be homeless for a month. My rental lease is up and I will have to stay in a hotel until I can find a place to live. My landlady had pulled a fast one on me; otherwise I'd have made better arrangements.

Needless to say, I am under a lot of duress in my personal life at the moment.

Several months ago, my psychiatric nurse practitioner prescribed Zoloft for me to combat my increasingly frequent anxiety attacks. Now, I have a history of anxiety and I used to take Xanax for 2 years, until I felt I didn't need it anymore. While packing my stuff I came across a bottle of four of these. And also a chocolate marijuana bar that a friend had given me, to try out and see if it would help with my recent bout of insomnia.

Marijuana is not legal in my state. Sure, it's legal for only glaucoma and some cancer patients, but there are no dispensaries, so this is still socially unacceptable here.

I eat the damn chocolate bar and boy did it help me sleep. I go into work 2 days later and all is OK.

I couldn't sleep again following this, so I take one of those old Xanax's. When I go into work the next day, I am disoriented, crying at my computer, and slurring my speech. The same Charge Nurse who's psych patient went AWOL? Well she orders me downstairs for a drug test. I didn't remember any of this happening. (The doctors later inform me that dissociation is a rare side effect of Zoloft, which I immediately stop taking).

Boom, I'm busted. THC and benzodiazepines, which I had not disclosed to the BON. The nightmare hospital fires me on the spot. I go home and call the Board to self-report.

In just a week's time I have become a low-down, dirty criminal.

I had taken a job at the other hospital closer to my house, the one I had applied for recently. I started my orientation and I need to say that I was so much happier here. This was also a post-op floor, but the floor was wonderfully managed.

Just when I get my anxiety down to a manageable level and start to fit in on this new floor, I get a thick letter from the BON stating that my license is now suspended.

Panic ensues and I don't know what to do. I had no idea they were gonna suspend my license, taking away my ability to work. Maybe submit me to random drug screens, outpatient rehab, sure. But suspend me?

My own nurse practitioner had trouble with the Board due to a DUI. They didn't suspend his license, but they made his life miserable for a few years. For 2 years, when he was still working as a floor nurse, he had to get the Charge Nurse to pull narcotics for him. I mean this was insane.

They do this overreach and excessive fines in the name of patient safety, and to some degree I can understand this. But nurses are patients too, aren't we?

I hired an attorney with what little money I had ($5,000), and submitted to an outpatient psych eval ($1,700). They ruled me safe to work, and that this was a one-time occurrence due to personal hardship... and to please reinstate my license. A panel of 3 experts submitted this report to the Board, that I had no history of drug abuse and was not a likely candidate for it. I don't know how they figure this stuff out, but they're experts and they have their ways. The evaluation was 10 hours long.

The brain acts very strangely when we're overly-stressed. Add exhaustion to that and the result is poor decision-making. I had had enough, passed my threshold, and I did something out of character. And for that I have had to remain jobless for a year and a half. Sure, I went to interview for other non-nursing jobs, but it always boiled down to not being able to make one of my random daytime drug screens.

My credit is now ruined because my student loans are so hefty. The Board "fines & fees" are excessive and unwarranted too, but that's the government nowadays. They have the power to do anything and there's not a damn thing any of us peons can do about it.

My contract with the Board was this: 2 years of random drug screens, continued outpatient rehab meetings with the addictionist there (I like this guy), and therapy on top of that.

After losing my application for reinstatement in January of this year, they finally got back to me and followed through with the promise. I was reinstated in April, 11 days short of a year since my license was suspended. I don't really have many restrictions, which I am grateful for. But I will be doing these random drug screens until November, 2016. This is why a regular day job has not been an option for me, and that is when my probation will end, and once again I will be "without restrictions & unencumbered."

I've had one job offer since my reinstatement regardless of my situation. I really loved this hospital. But for reasons unknown, they have since withdrawn the offer.

I am currently still interviewing and applying for work. I suffered my second miscarriage in October. I haven't gotten my period since March.

But I have become very numb to the depression.

I guess when you hit rock bottom like I did, there is only one place left to go: back up.

* * *

Things You Should Know Before Hitting the Floor

March, 2015

If you're taking *any* medications or have any conditions like diagnosed anxiety, let the BON know. If you don't and they find out, they will suspend your license on the grounds of "Failure to Disclose." Even for dental work & child birth, if you have to take narcotics even for a few days, notify the BON. Telling only your employer will not suffice.

If you're taking a medication that was prescribed to you two years prior, it's legally no longer your medication (and it's probably expired).

Make sure you have liability/malpractice insurance upon graduation. It's only $108 per year with NSO, and in the event that something should happen to you (i.e. a patient sues the hospital, or if you screw up), this will cover a lawyer's fee and you will have saved thousands, possibly more.

Unless you know somebody, your first year working as a nurse will have you regretting the choice you've made. Don't give in to this sentiment. It gets much better.

Give up alcohol (& drugs if you did them before), unless you don't mind risking all that you've worked for. One DUI will give you *years* of misery with the BON. I don't have this myself, but I know several nurses who do.

Upon your first few interviews, if you get a nagging feeling about a floor, don't work there. Trust your instincts. Look at the nurses' faces. Do they look frantic, miserable? Never take a job on a floor that bleeds nurses. If you have to, then just keep applying for jobs and leave the miserable place once a new offer is made to you. It doesn't matter if you've only got 2 or 3 months of experience. Jump on the new offer & leave the toxic place behind.

Getting your BLS & ACLS on your own will not improve your chances of being hired. Whoever hires you will have someone who can certify you in a day, and you'll save $200.

Fluency in another language will not (usually) improve your chances of getting hired. If you're working on a floor where the doctors are constantly requesting that you translate (even knowing you're not certified), thus snatching you away from *your* patients, then ask for a pay raise. They won't honor this.

If you're not a social critter or if you have bad nerves, then work toward landing a job on night shift or in the ICU. You will enjoy nursing so much more when you're in your element & can actually hear yourself think.

Kill 'em with kindness. Nurses & other employees with bad attitudes will make a new nurse more anxious. It'll hurt you none to be kind to people who haven't gotten to know you yet. You never know what's going on in their lives to make them act that way. It'll be several months of hard adjustment once you graduate, but it won't be this way forever. Besides, who the hell cares what they think? It's not like they're paying your bills.

* * *

Life After the Fall

August, 2015

Finally I've found a job.

It's been two months now since I began and I'm now out of orientation. This is at a hospital 30 minutes from my house. It's a big hospital and, even though its reputation is shady, turned out to be a good work environment. It's not in the inner-city & doesn't boast all the miracles that the nightmare hospital did.

I took a night shift position on a Medicine floor, which means a wide array of illnesses, but not half as much pain. And maybe it's because it is a night shift job that I like it so much more. There are hardly any visitors during the night, no tests to send my patients to, no physical therapy, no dietary issues I have to deal with.

Of course, it's not where I wanted to be. I'd like to specialize in *something* one day. But I can see myself working here for a long time, and until my student loans are paid off, this is all that matters.

I often think about what happened to me. I own up to it. It was completely my fault. But I still have a problem with hospitals that put their nurses in awkward situations.

At first I thought I was an incompetent nurse. I mean, I felt this way all throughout nursing school, as did pretty much all the other new nurses. But I've learned something from that first job. At least now I can tell the difference between an incompetent nurse and an incompetent management. I won't ever get this confused again. When every nurse on the floor has a list of complaints and things do not change, it's time to go elsewhere.

I'm still not 100% and I'm learning new things every week. So far my co-workers and patients have been great. Because of this, I'm not throwing up every time I get in the car & drive to work. I'm not contemplating the bad things that can happen. Sure, sometimes they do. But this is to be expected in the medical field. In any field.

I'm at a good balance right now, where I can handle every single thing that is thrown my way, the way I was trained. It's not like it was before. That nightmare was impossible. Impossible for anyone to last in. Because of this change in my life, I am now more confident in myself.

Throughout this whole ordeal I was convinced that all the other nurses were so much stronger than me. Then I think about the seasoned nurse who'd go home every day & hit the bottle. I never did this. I mean, the one time I did do something *like* this, I was caught.

My brother tells me that it was for the better, but I'm not so sure.

Would I have otherwise gone on to be a drug addict, and worse, kill my patient?

So maybe he is right.

I feel as though I am a lot stronger than I once was. There were times when I felt that I'd be better off dead. But every time I'd go interview and tell them about my situation, they'd understand. They were so warm about it, and would tell me stories of worse things happening to nurses they knew.

And I loved this about them.

This is the stuff that makes a nurse: warmth & compassion. I get it now. And I remind myself every day that these are two attributes I'm not lacking in. This is how I make my patients feel.

This was why I became a nurse.